miracle juices™

detox

Safety Note

Detox should not be considered a replacement for professional medical treatment; a physician should be consulted on all matters relating to health. While the advice and information in this book is believed to be accurate, the publisher cannot accept any legal responsibility or liability for any injury or illness sustained while following the advice in this book.

First published in Great Britain in 2002 by Hamlyn,
a division of Octopus Publishing Group Ltd
2–4 Heron Quays, London E14 4JP

ISBN 0 600 60674 0

A CIP catalogue record for this book is available from the British Library

Printed and bound in China

10 9 8 7 6 5 4 3 2 1

Contents

introduction

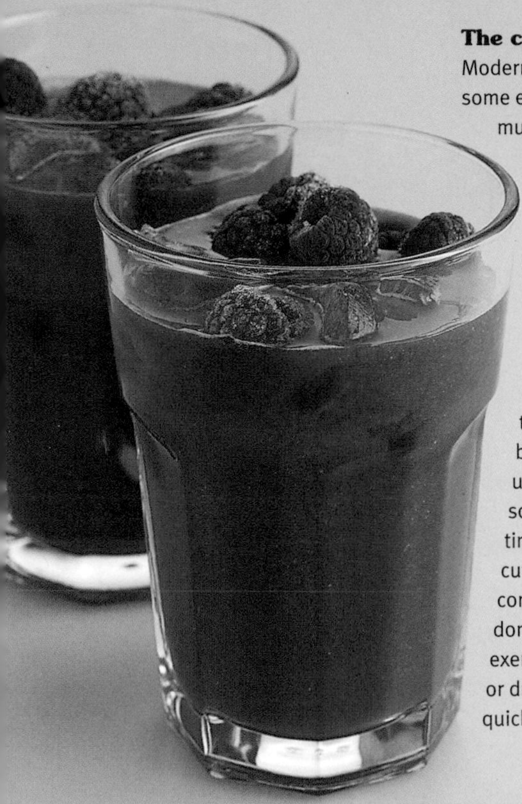

The case for detox

Modern life is necessarily toxic to some extent. Every day we face a multitude of pollutants and chemicals in the air that we breathe and in the food and water we consume. In addition, we tend to run our lives at an incredible pace – we have demanding, stressful jobs that may involve long hours of travelling, we run homes, bring up children and usually try to fit in hectic social lives, too. Because time is short, we invariably cut corners. We eat convenience or junk food, we don't get enough sleep or exercise and we often smoke or drink too much alcohol as a quick-fix way to relax.

The body treats all the toxins it encounters as a matter of urgency and works on processing them to render them harmless, or 'detoxed'. This leaves less energy for the everyday processes of cleansing, healing and renewal. Over time, the body can't keep up the pace, the strain shows on the overworked liver and kidneys and the body's performance slows down. The effects of this slow-down and the build-up of toxins emerge in many different forms – everything from continual fatigue, passing infections, skin eruptions, headaches and digestive problems to serious conditions, such as ulcers, cancer and heart disease.

How detox works

A detoxification diet allows two things to happen. First, by abstaining from certain foods we stop overloading the body with harmful substances and, secondly, we give it plenty of the right nutrients to actually speed up the elimination of old toxins and unwanted waste and promote cell renewal. As the cells are rejuvenated, your body becomes healthier and you look and feel younger! As well as losing any excess weight, you can expect to have clear skin, healthy-looking hair, strong nails and lots more energy. Detoxing also has a very calming effect on the mind, particularly if you combine it with a relaxation technique, such as yoga or meditation.

Detoxification need not involve only diet. There are various external treatments that can work alongside a detox diet to help the general detox process. These include facial exfoliation, hydrotherapy, skin brushing and manual lymphatic drainage massage.

detox guidelines

A detoxification programme is ideal if you have been over-indulging and feel lethargic, listless and bloated. Don't attempt a lengthy detox programme, which you may break early out of sheer hunger. Instead, try a weekend-long detox plan, or even a one-day juice plan (see pages 8–9), and concentrate on drinking juices that speed up the detox process and aid digestion and the immune system. A one-day detox can be repeated every week if you wish.

Since much of the nutritional value of food is lost in its cooking and processing, uncooked fresh produce with its high vitamin and mineral content is at the core of any detox plan. A one-day detox plan consists entirely of freshly made fruit and vegetable juices, which help cleanse the blood and tissues of toxins and regenerate the entire system. Organic fresh produce is preferable so that you don't replace some of the toxins you are eliminating with pesticide residues.

A longer detox programme involves several stages, starting with liquids only, then gradually adding raw fruits and vegetables, cooked vegetables and brown rice, grains and live yogurts, and finally fish. After any period of consuming liquids only you must return to food slowly or you will overload the digestive system, undo all you have achieved and even feel unwell.

Do not detox if you:

- **are underweight**
- **are pregnant or breast-feeding**
- **have anaemia**
- **have Type 1 diabetes**
- **are following a course of prescription medication**
- **have kidney failure**
- **have severe liver disease**

During detoxification, side effects such as tiredness, muscle pains, mood swings, headaches and skin problems are inevitable as the toxins make their way out. However, do persevere — within a relatively short time you will feel re-energized and rejuvenated, and have better-looking skin, hair and nails.

After detox

By eliminating the substances that are harmful to your body — in particular caffeine, nicotine, alcohol, over-the-counter drugs (but check with your doctor about prescribed drugs) and processed carbohydrates and sugars — your body will feel lighter and less bloated. Continue the good work after detoxing by keeping your intake of these substances moderate or banishing them from your diet altogether and replacing them with healthy alternatives.

one-day detox plan

A one-day juice detox is beneficial for two reasons. You'll be clearing your body of a build-up of toxins, which could be contributing to certain ailments. Also, although you may feel slightly tired or headachy as your body goes without sugars or caffeine, it should be a day dedicated solely to

8.00 am	Drink a glass of warm water with a little lemon juice to help flush out the kidneys.
8.30 am	Make a juice with a little citrus fruit in it, or apple, pineapple or melon (see Ultimate Detox, page 18, Berry Booster, page 38 or Juice Boost, page 62) to wake you up and begin the cleansing process.
9.00 am	Get your circulation moving with dry skin brushing to stimulate the circulatory and lymphatic systems. Using a natural bristle brush, begin at your feet, and with long, smooth movements gently move upwards. Finish with a warm shower then a blast of cold water if you're feeling brave! Dry yourself and moisturize your skin.
9.30 am	Have a glass of water or a herbal tea which will aid the detox process.
10.00 am	Take a gentle walk or swim or try a yoga class. By moving your body, you're less likely to feel the side effects of a detox, such as tiredness or headaches, and you'll also be helping your body rid itself of toxins.
11.30 am	After exercising, have another glass of water or a herbal tea.
12.30 pm	At lunchtime, choose a filling juice to alleviate hunger pains. Try a combination of root vegetables and leafy greens (*see* Magnificent 7, page 20 or Squeaky Green, page 56).
1.00pm	Have another glass of water or a herbal tea — ginger is good for the stomach, while lemon is a good tea for detoxification.

you, to relax and rejuvenate. Try not to arrange any appointments and, if you want to exercise, don't do anything too strenuous. Do something you enjoy, whether it's reading, relaxing or having a lie-in. There are no hard and fast rules for a one-day detox, just spend the day looking after yourself.

1.30pm A detox programme can be quite tiring, as your body is ridding itself of a build-up of toxins. Have a nap or lie down and read or listen to some relaxing music.

2.30pm Have another glass of water or a herbal tea.

3.30pm Your blood sugar levels may be feeling a little low by now, so you can pack this juice full of fruits such as blueberries, strawberries, cranberries, oranges and mangoes. It may taste slightly tart after a relatively food-free day, but you'll feel energized afterwards.

5.00pm It's important to drink at least eight glasses of water every day, so have another glass now.

7.30pm You'll probably have no problems going to sleep tonight, but make a juice that contains ingredients such as bananas, lettuce or apples to aid relaxation and beat insomnia (*see* Fig Feast, page 28 or Sleep Tight, page 46).

9.30pm Have another glass of water and then your last herbal tea, a calming one before bedtime, such as chamomile tea. Have a relaxing bath, adding aromatherapy oils such as lavender, ylang ylang, rose or sandalwood.

10.00pm Bedtime. Your stomach will be relatively empty by tomorrow morning, so start the day gradually with some fresh fruit and yogurt or wholemeal toast and honey. Opt for a light salad lunch, and possibly some steamed vegetables and rice for dinner, supplemented of course by a couple of fresh nutritious juices.

why juice?

Vital vitamins and minerals such as antioxidants, vitamins A, B, C and E, folic acid, potassium, calcium, magnesium, zinc and amino acids are present in fresh fruits and vegetables, and are all necessary for optimum health. Because juicing removes the indigestible fibre in fruits and vegetables, the nutrients are available to the body in much larger quantities than if the piece of fruit or vegetable were eaten whole. For example, when you eat a raw carrot you are able to assimilate only about 1 per cent of the available beta-carotene, because many of the nutrients are trapped in the fibre. When a carrot is juiced, thereby removing the fibre, nearly 100 per cent of the beta-carotene can be assimilated. Juicing several types of fruits and vegetables on a daily basis is therefore an easy way to ensure that your body receives its full quota of vitamins and minerals.

In addition, fruits and vegetables provide another substance absolutely essential for good health — water. Most people don't consume enough water. In fact, many of the fluids we drink — coffee, tea, soft drinks, alcoholic beverages and artificially flavoured drinks — contain substances that require extra water for the body to eliminate, and tend to be dehydrating. Fruit and vegetable juices are free of these unnecessary substances.

Your health

A diet high in fruits and vegetables can prevent and help to cure a wide range of ailments. At the cutting edge of nutritional research are the plant chemicals known as phytochemicals, which hold the key to preventing deadly diseases such as cancer and heart disease, and others such as asthma, arthritis and allergies.

Although juicing benefits your overall health, it should be used only to complement your daily eating plan. You must still eat enough from the other food groups (such as grains, dairy food and pulses) to ensure your body maintains strong bones and healthy cells. If you are following a specially prescribed diet, or are under medical supervision, do discuss any drastic changes with your health practitioner before beginning any type of new health regime.

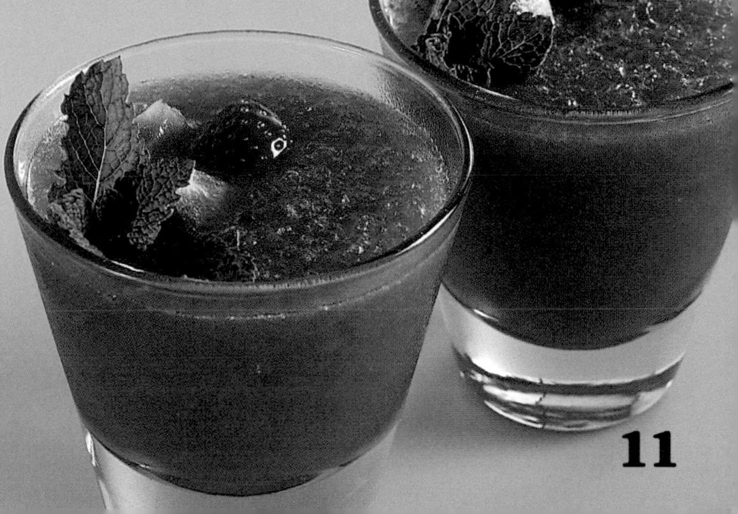

how to juice

Available in a variety of models, juicers work by separating the fruit and vegetable juice from the pulp. Choose a juicer with a reputable brand name, that has an opening big enough for larger fruits and vegetables, and make sure it is easy to take apart and clean, otherwise you may become discouraged from using it.

Types of juicer

A citrus juicer or lemon squeezer is ideal for extracting the juice from oranges, lemons, limes and grapefruit, especially if you want to add just a small amount of citrus juice to another liquid. Pure citrus juice has a high acid content, which may upset your stomach, so it is best diluted.

Centrifugal juicers are the most widely used and affordable juicers available. Fresh fruits and vegetables are fed into a rapidly spinning grater, and the pulp separated from the juice by centrifugal force. The pulp is retained in the machine while the juice runs into a separate jug. A centrifugal juicer produces less juice than the more expensive masticating juicer, which works by pulverizing fruits and vegetables, and pushing them through a wire mesh with immense force.

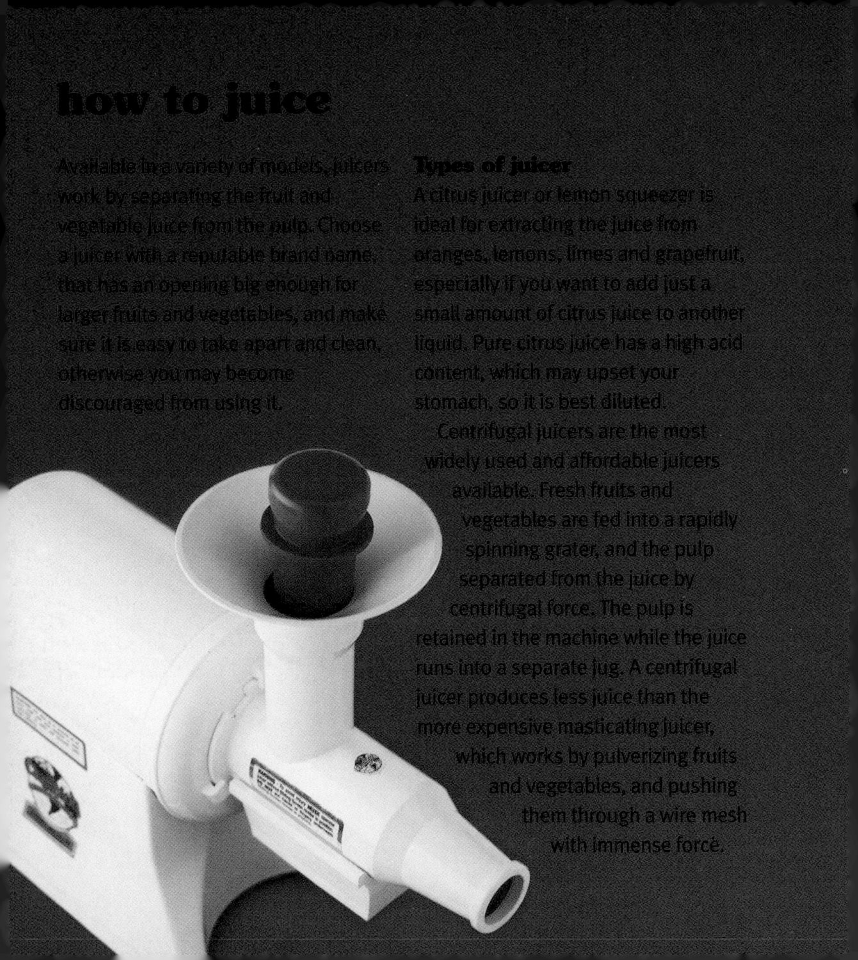

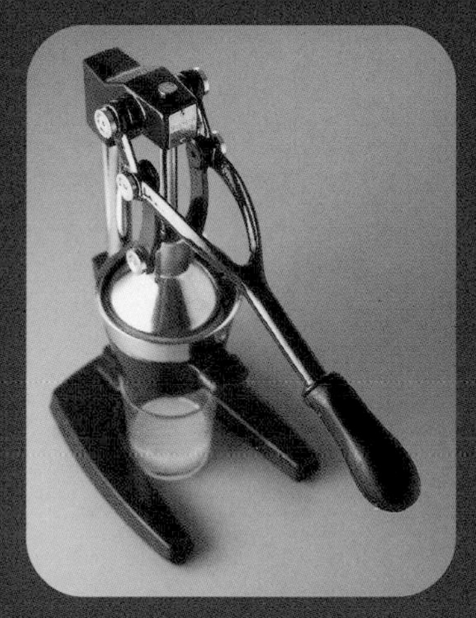

Cleaning the juicer

Clean your juicing machine thoroughly, as any residue left may harbour bacterial growth — a toothbrush or nailbrush works well for removing stubborn residual pulp. Leaving the equipment to soak in warm soapy water will loosen the residue from those hard-to-reach places. A solution made up of one part white vinegar to two parts water will lessen any staining produced by the fruits and vegetables.

Preparing produce for juicing

It is best to prepare ingredients just before juicing so that fewer nutrients are lost through oxidization. Cut or tear foods into manageable pieces for juicing. If the ingredients are not organic, do not include stems, skins or roots, but if the produce is organic, you can put everything in the juicer. However, don't include the skins from pineapple, mango, papaya, citrus fruit and banana, and remove the stones from avocados, apricots, peaches, mangoes and plums. You can include melon seeds, particularly watermelon, as these are full of juice. For grape juice, choose green grapes with an amber tinge or black grapes with a darkish bloom. Leave the pith on lemons for the pectin content.

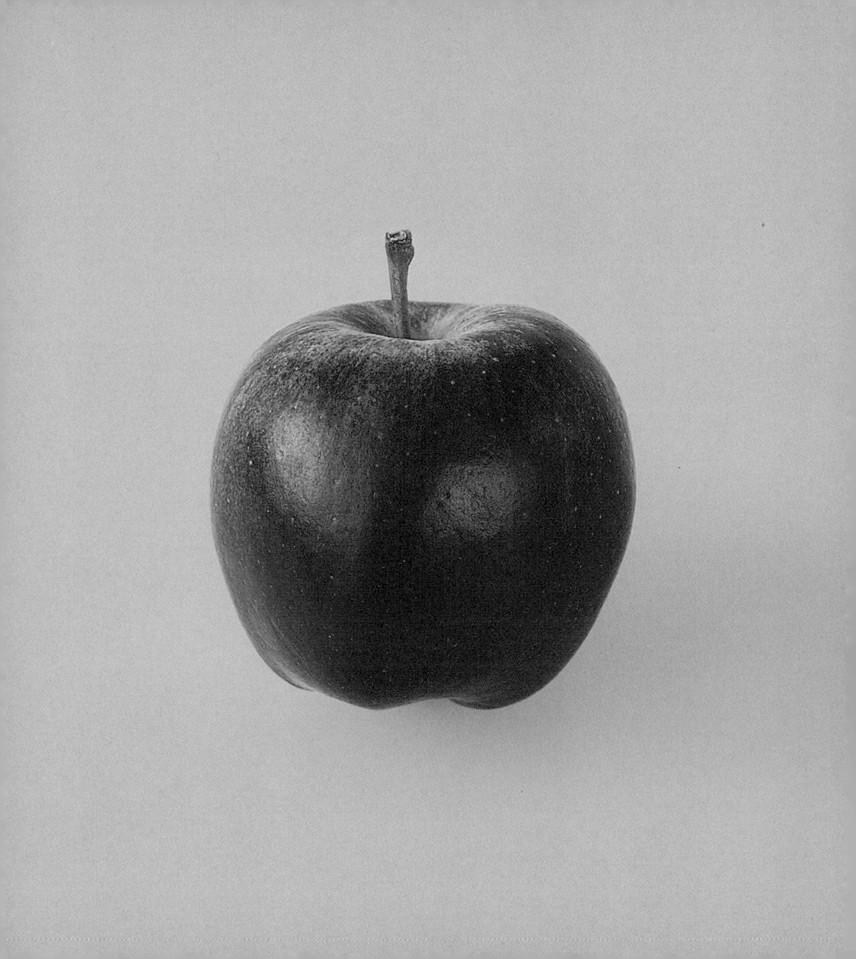

eliminate

A good detox juice, this ultra green juice helps to maintain energy levels. Leafy green vegetables are particularly good for an overtaxed liver. Parsley is a mild diuretic and contains zinc and trace minerals that aid liver function, while celery helps cleanse the liver and lymph system and aids digestion.

green peace

100 g (3½ oz) broccoli
100 g (3½ oz) kale
25 g (1 oz) parsley
200 g (7 oz) apple
50 g (2 oz) celery

Juice all the ingredients and serve in a glass over ice. Decorate with kale, if liked.
Makes 200 ml (7 fl oz)

Nutritional Values

- Kcals 228
- Vitamin A 10574 iu
- Vitamin C 365 mg
- Selenium 5.14 mcg
- Zinc 1 mg

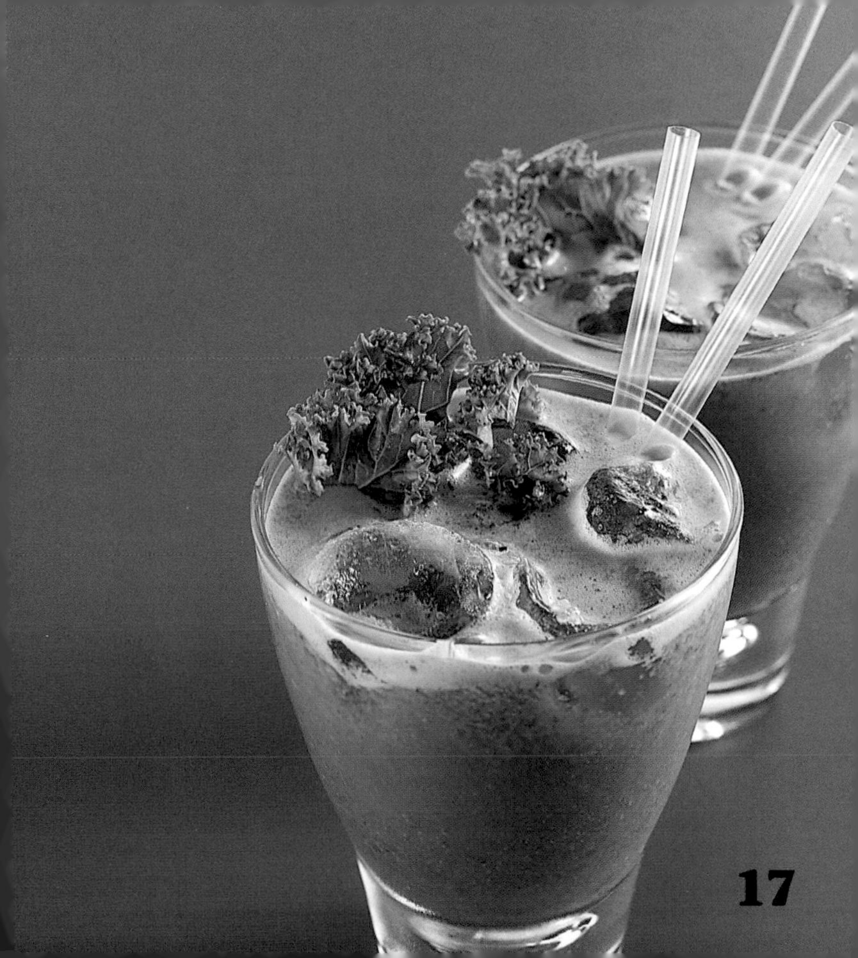

Simply delicious, this juice is the best general tonic for internal cleansing and for boosting the immune system. Both apples and carrots are exceptionally high in minerals and vitamins and are great cleansers.

ultimate detox

4 carrots
2 green apples

Juice both the ingredients and serve in a tall glass over ice. Decorate with slices of apple, if liked.

Makes 300 ml (½ pint)

Nutritional Values

- Kcals 280
- Vitamin A 80356 iu
- Vitamin C 44 mg
- Potassium 1280 mg

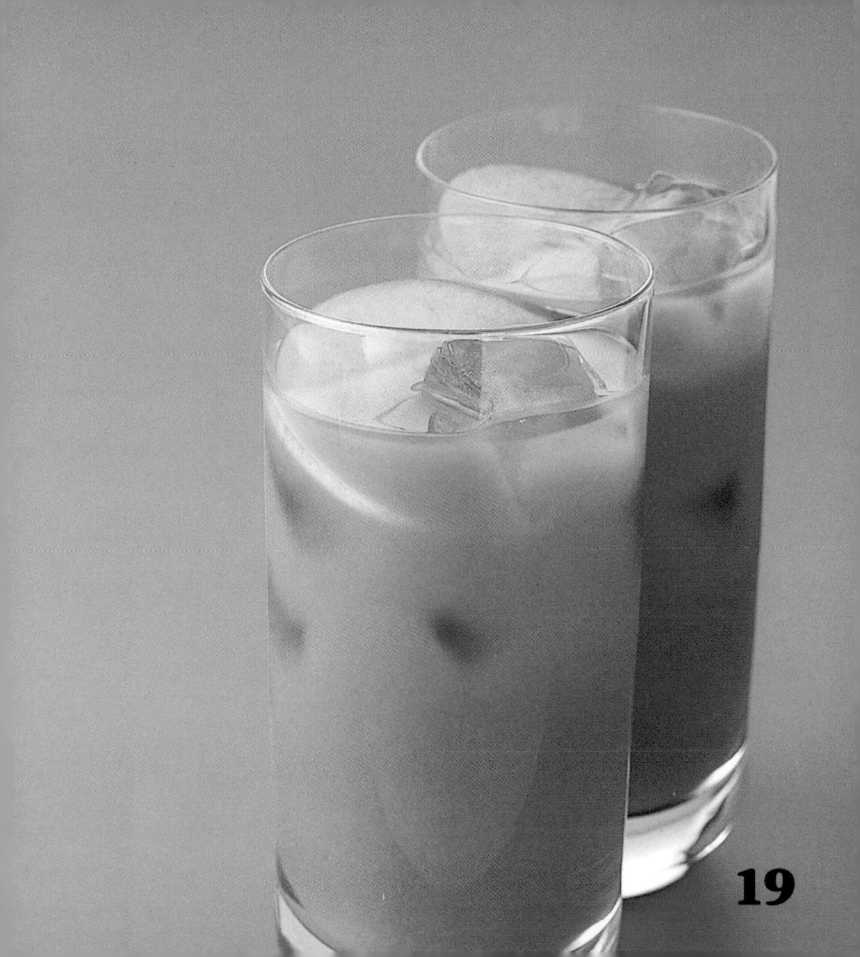

A great all-round energy booster, this juice acts as a diuretic, helping flush out the harmful elements in your system and boosting vitamin levels.

magnificent 7

90 g (3 oz) carrot
50 g (2 oz) green pepper
25 g (1 oz) spinach
25 g (1 oz) onion
50 g (2 oz) celery
90 g (3 oz) cucumber
50 g (2 oz) tomato
sea salt and pepper

Juice all the ingredients and season with sea salt and pepper to taste. Serve over ice and decorate with tomato quarters, if liked.

Makes 200 ml (7 fl oz)

Nutritional Values

- Kcals 115
- Vitamin A 28009 iu
- Vitamin C 105 mg
- Iron 2.41 mg
- Potassium 1065 mg
- Selenium 2.5 mcg
- Zinc 0.8 mg

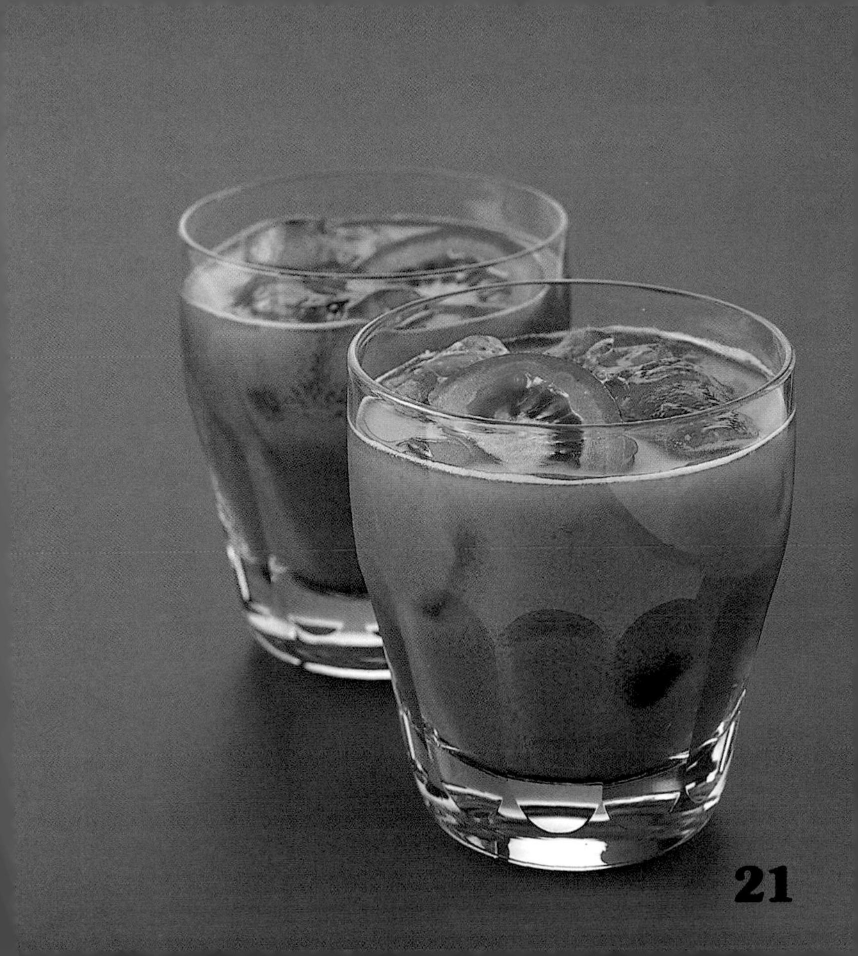

A diuretic, watermelon speeds the passage of fluids carrying toxins through the system. The seeds are full of juice and can be juiced too, if liked.

water baby

¼ watermelon, about 300 g (10 oz) flesh
125 g (4 oz) raspberries

Remove the skin from the watermelon and chop the flesh into even-sized pieces. Juice the watermelon and raspberries, pour into a large glass and add a couple of ice cubes. Decorate with raspberries, if liked.

Makes 350 ml (12 fl oz)

Nutritional Values

- Kcals 125
- Vitamin A 1330 iu
- Vitamin C 60 mg
- Potassium 559 mg
- Iron 1.8 mg
- Calcium 52 mg

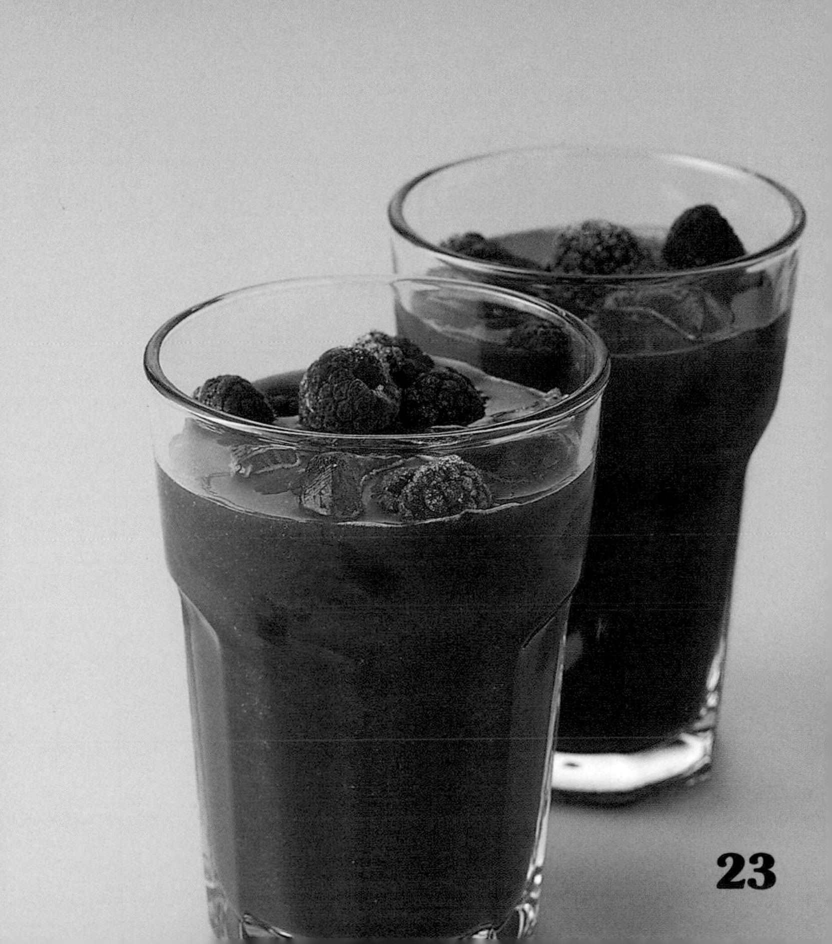
23

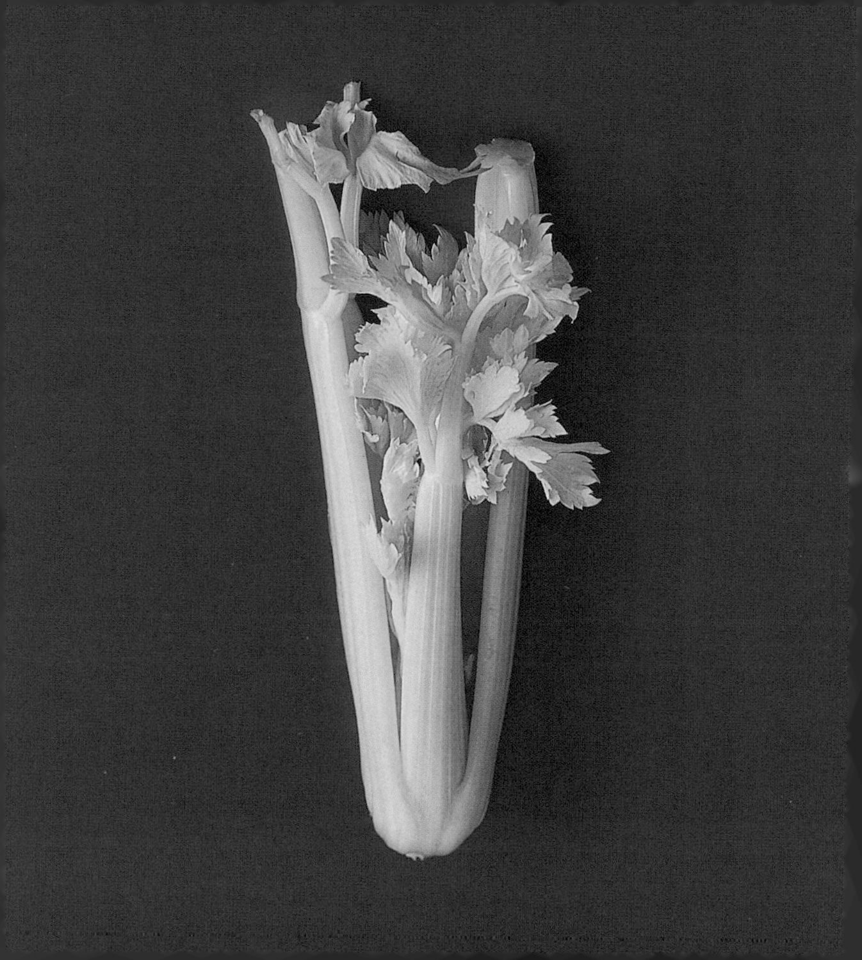

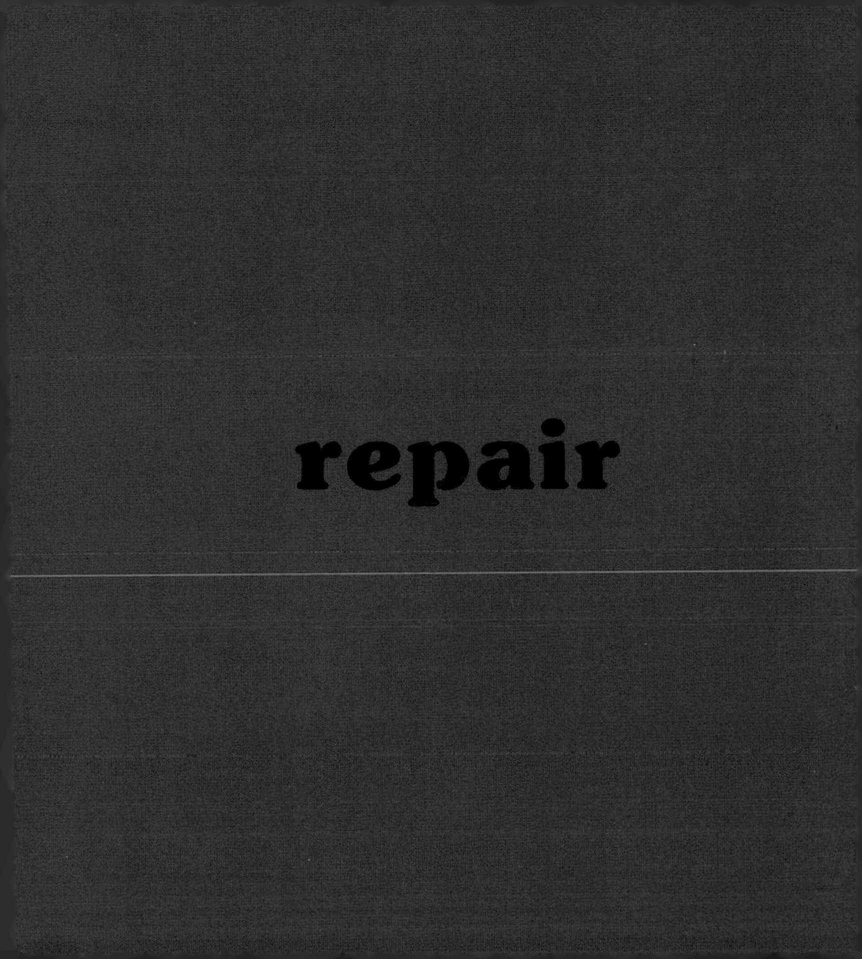
repair

The cucumber in this juice provides protective antioxidants for the digestive tract and, together with the melon and cranberries, acts as a diuretic to cleanse the intestinal system.

flush-a-bye-baby

250 g (8 oz) cranberries
250 g (8 oz) watermelon or galia melon, peeled
250 g (8 oz) cucumber

Juice all the ingredients, including the pips of the melon and the skin of the cucumber. Serve in a tumbler and decorate with melon sticks, if liked.
Makes 200 ml (7 fl oz)

Nutritional Values

- Kcals 232
- Vitamin A 8475 iu
- Vitamin C 120 mg
- Potassium 880 mg
- Iron 4.7 mg
- Calcium 92.5 mg

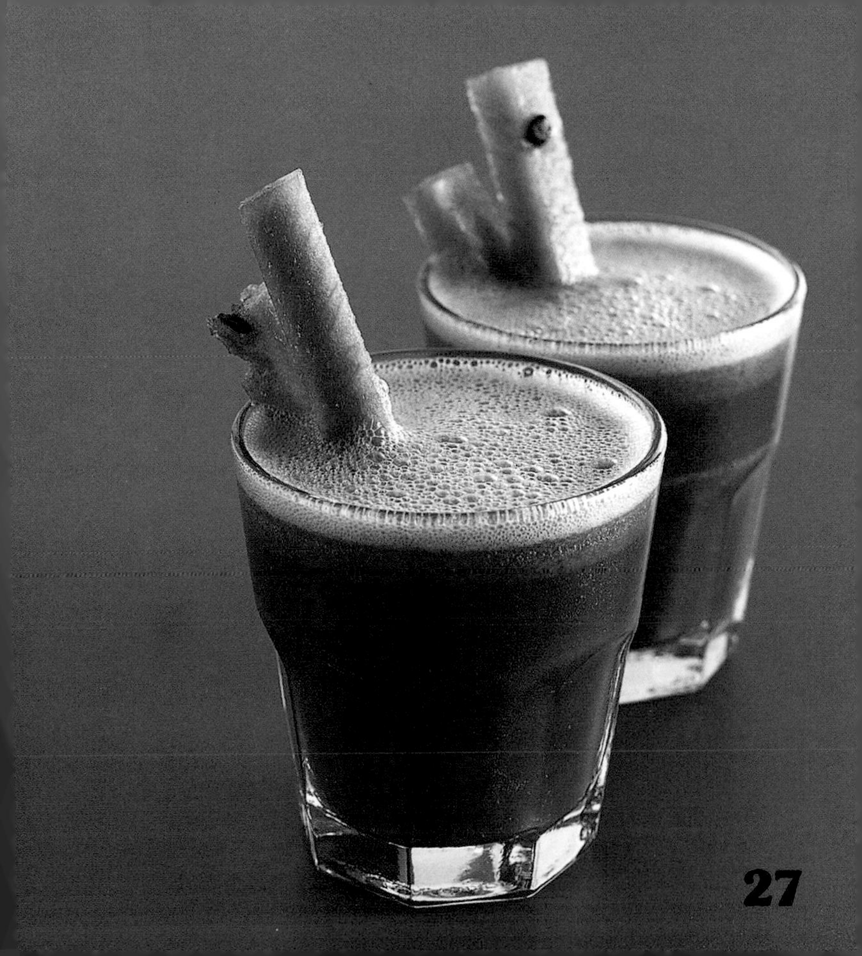

Bananas and figs are rich in tryptophan. This is converted in the body into the brain chemical serotonin, which can induce a feeling of wellbeing. Because these fruits are high in natural sugars they produce a feeling of fullness, which can help stave off hunger if you are on a juice-only detox plan.

fig feast

250 g (8 oz) carrot
100 g (3½ oz) figs
1 orange, peeled
2.5 cm (1 inch) cube of fresh root ginger, roughly chopped
100 g (3½ oz) peeled banana

Juice the carrot, figs, orange and ginger. Put the juice into a blender with the banana and a couple of ice cubes and whizz for 20 seconds for a delicious smoothie. Add more ice cubes and decorate with sliced figs, if liked.
Makes 200 ml (7 fl oz)

Nutritional Values

- Kcals 460
- Vitamin A 14117 iu
- Vitamin B6 0.23 mg
- Vitamin C 192 mg
- Magnesium 118 mg
- Tryptophan 89 mg

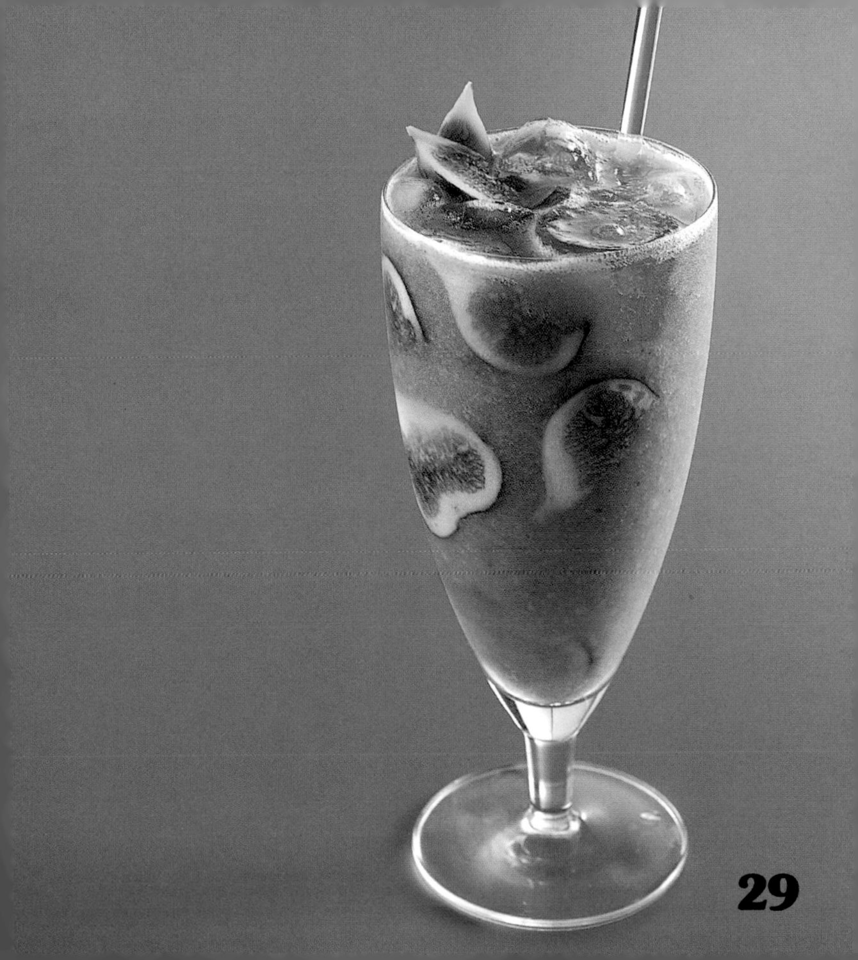

Cabbage is a great detoxifier. It aids digestion and prevents fluid retention and constipation. Cabbage is perfect for juicing as its nutrients are most abundant when it is eaten raw. Celery, watercress and pears are the ideal accompaniments as they also contribute to the detoxification process. Watercress is a powerful intestinal cleanser, the cabbage and the pear rid the colon of waste matter and the celery purifies the lymph.

spring clean

250 g (8 oz) pear
125 g (4 oz) cabbage
50 g (2 oz) celery
25 g (1 oz) watercress

Juice all the ingredients and serve over ice, decorated with celery sticks, if liked.
Makes 200 ml (7 fl oz)

Nutritional Values

- Kcals 206
- Vitamin C 97 mg
- Potassium 1129 mg
- Magnesium 48 mg

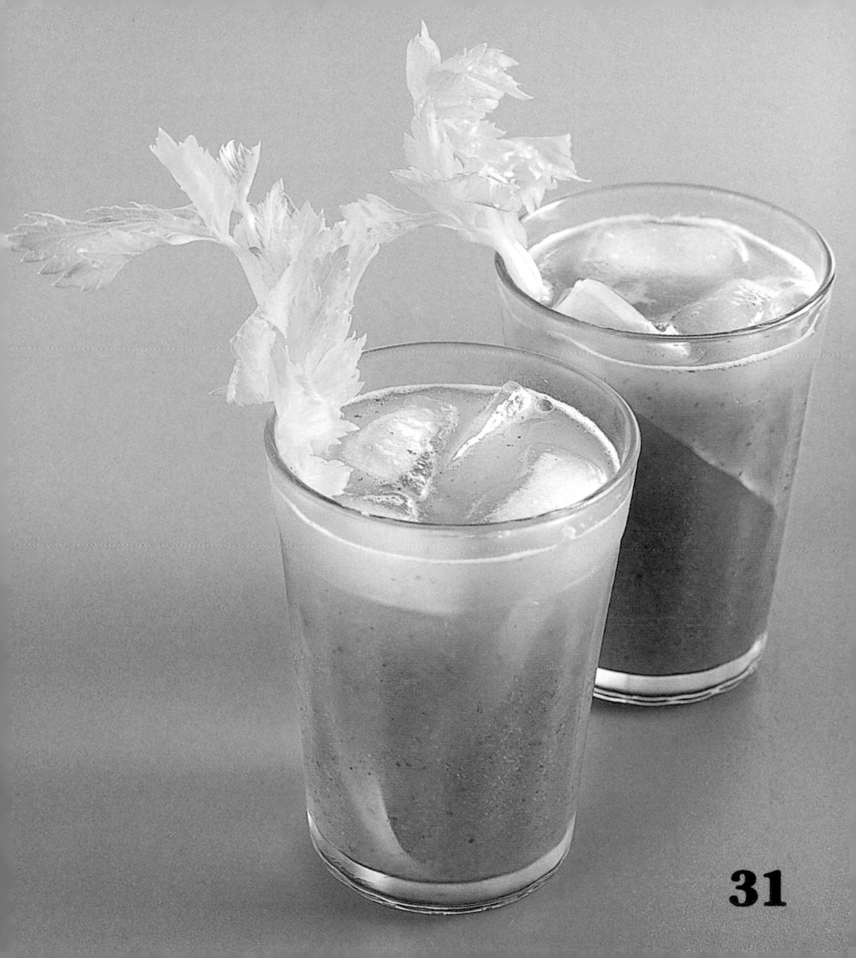

31

This juice is particularly good for the skin, which as the body's largest organ of elimination is the barometer of health and therefore the first to show any imbalances. Encouragingly, the skin is also the first part of the body to show the positive results of detoxifying your system.

herbi-four

175 g (6 oz) red pepper
175 g (6 oz) tomatoes
100 g (3½ oz) white cabbage
1 tablespoon chopped parsley

Juice the red pepper, tomatoes and cabbage. Pour into a tall glass over ice, stir in the parsley and decorate with thin wedges of lime, if liked.

Makes 200 ml (7 fl oz)

Nutritional Values

- Kcals 120
- Vitamin A 4062 iu
- Vitamin C 264 mg
- Selenium 2.13 mcg
- Zinc 1.14 mg

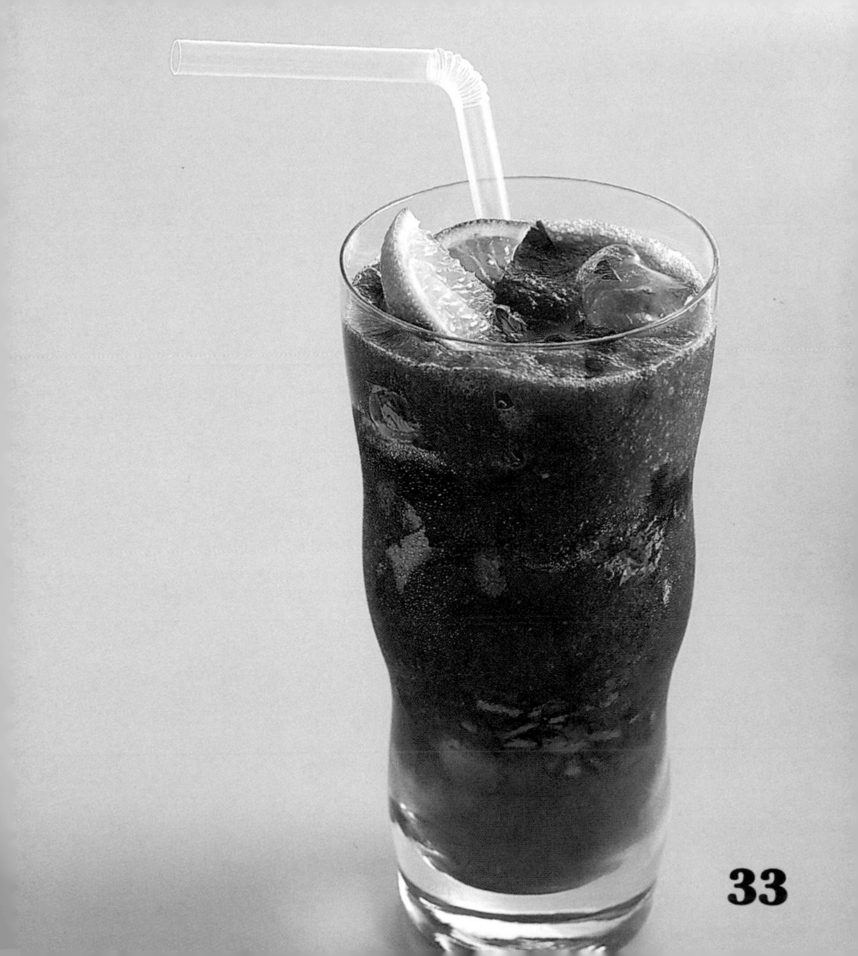
33

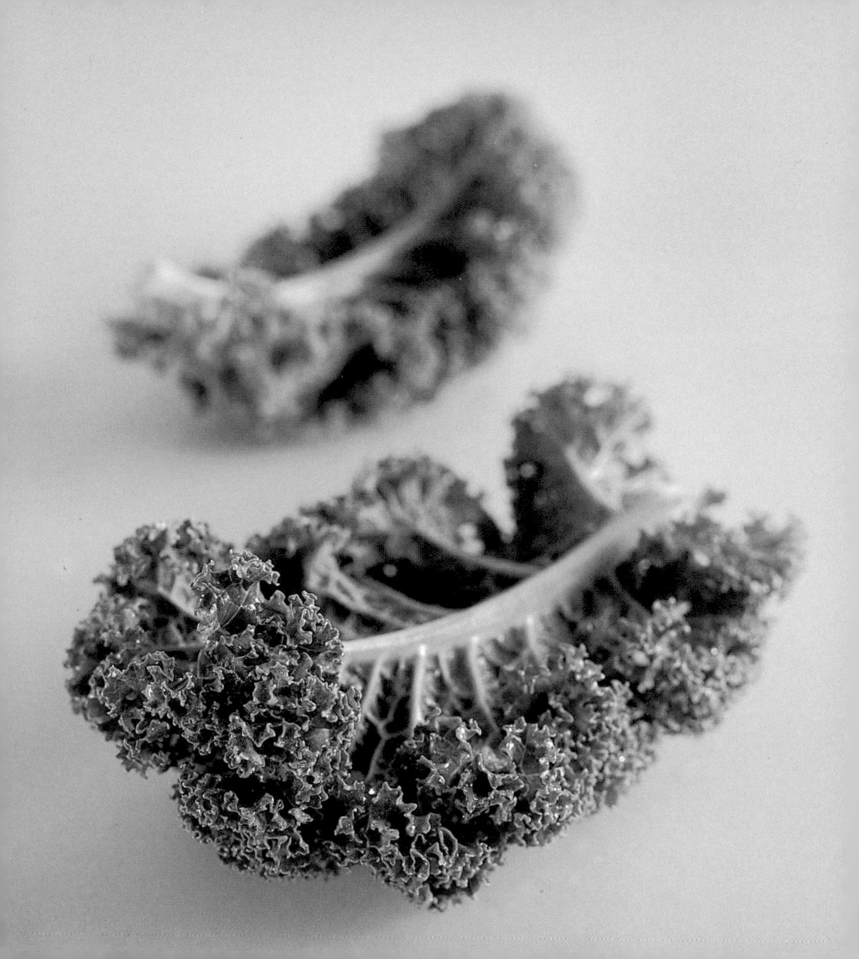

cleanse

A sharp, clean-tasting drink full of vitamins A and C, selenium and zinc, this juice is an excellent internal cleanser.

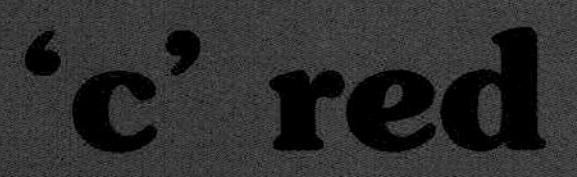

150 g (5 oz) grapefruit
50 g (2 oz) kiwi fruit
175 g (6 oz) pineapple
50 g (2 oz) frozen raspberries
50 g (2 oz) frozen cranberries

Juice the grapefruit, kiwi fruit and pineapple. Whizz in a blender with the frozen berries. Decorate with raspberries, if liked.

Makes 200 ml (7 fl oz)

Nutritional Values

- Kcals 247
- Vitamin A 693 iu
- Vitamin C 179 mg
- Selenium 4.3 mcg
- Zinc 1.43 mg

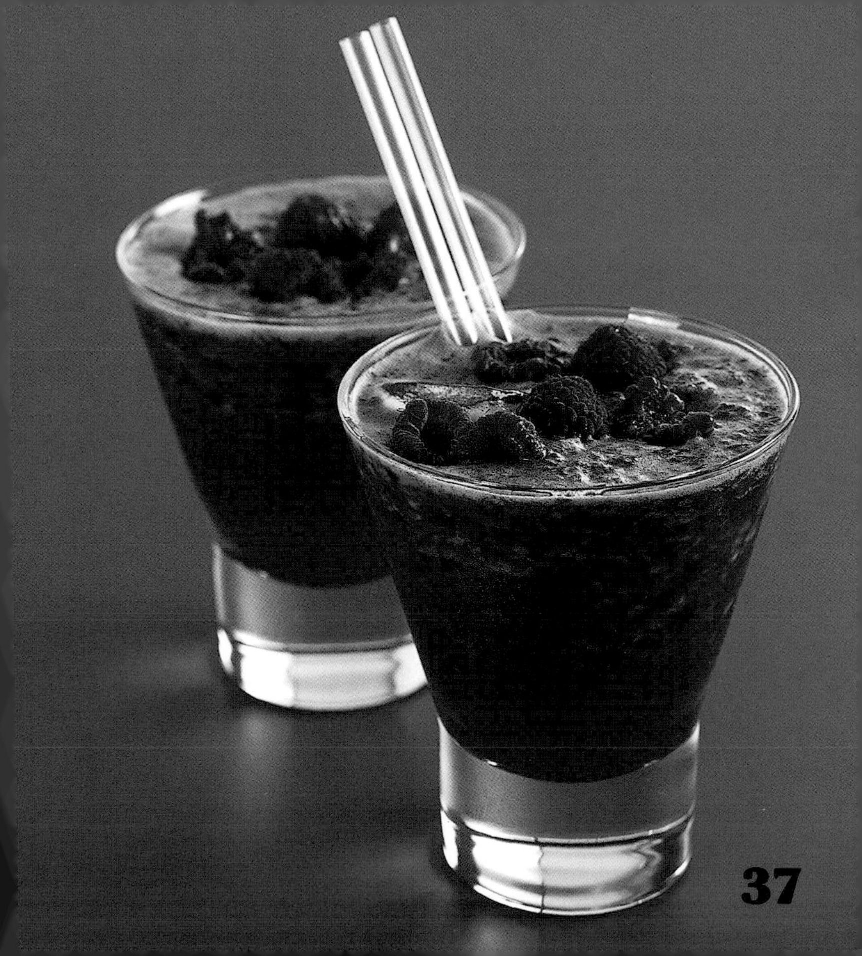

The enzyme bromelin, which is found in pineapple, helps the digestive system by encouraging the growth of 'good' bacteria in the gut at the expense of bad bacteria. Blackberries are good for the immune system.

berry booster

375 g (12 oz) blackberries
375 g (12 oz) pineapple flesh or 1 small pineapple, peeled

Juice the blackberries first, then the pineapple, to push through the pulp. Blend the juice with a couple of ice cubes and serve in a tall glass, decorated with a sliver of pineapple, if liked.
Makes 200 ml (7 fl oz)

Nutritional Values

- Kcals 353
- Vitamin A 658 iu
- Vitamin C 129.5 mg
- Iron 3.29 mg
- Potassium 1081 mg
- Calcium 136 mg
- Folic acid 340 mcg

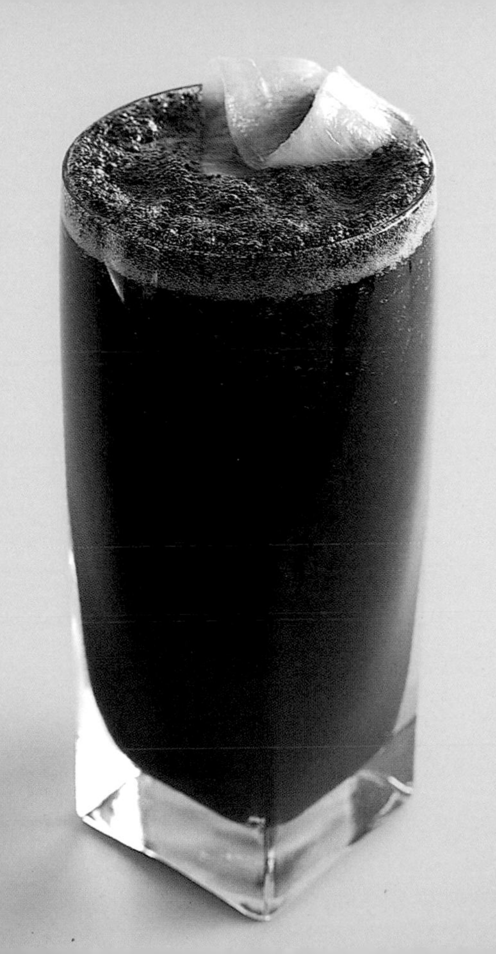

39

This is a particularly good juice to drink after exercise. The cucumber flushes out the kidneys and the grapefruit aids the elimination of toxins.

lemon aid

625 g (1¼ lb) grapefruit flesh
750 g (1½ lb) cucumber
1 lemon, peeled
sparkling mineral water, to top up

Juice the grapefruit, cucumber and lemon. Pour into a jug over ice, and top up with sparkling mineral water. Pour into glasses and decorate with sprigs of mint and slices of lemon, if liked.

Makes 400 ml (14 fl oz)

Nutritional Values

- Kcals 302
- Vitamin C 273 mg
- Potassium 1627 mg
- Magnesium 1332 mg
- Zinc 1.9 mg

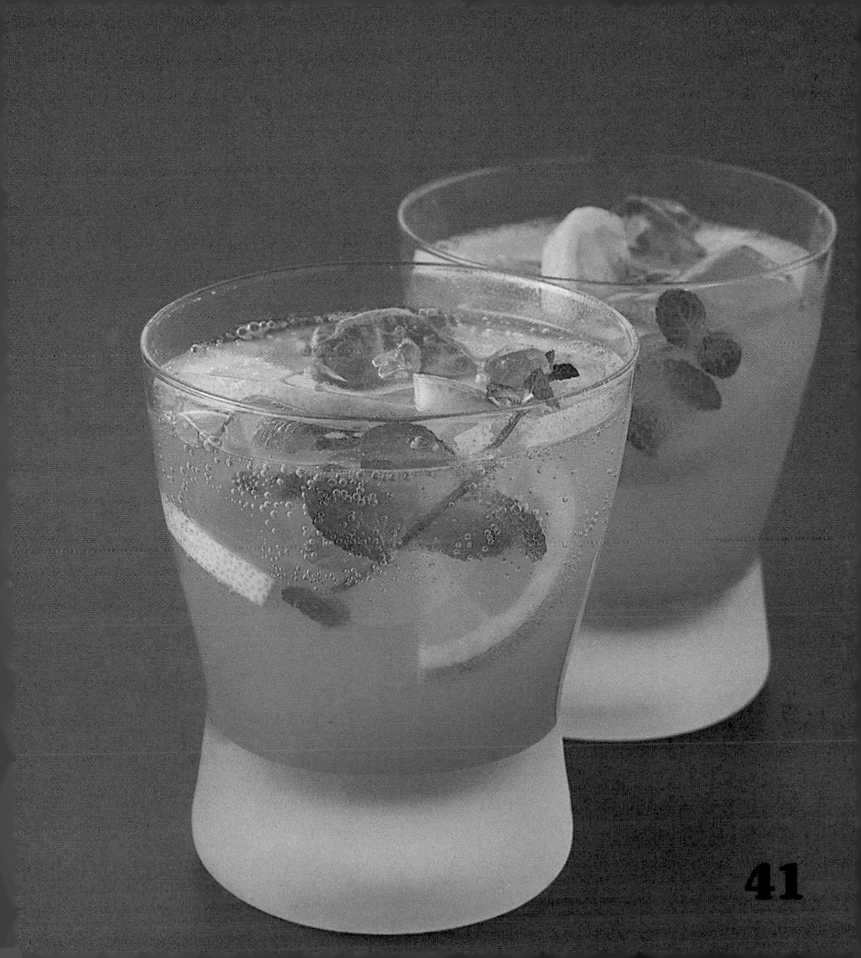

Carrot and apple contain pectin, tannic acid and malic acid, which help regulate bowel movement and soothe intestinal walls. Cabbage detoxifies the stomach and upper colon and improves the digestion.

system soother

175 g (6 oz) carrot
250 g (8 oz) apple
125 g (4 oz) red cabbage

Juice all the ingredients, including the apple cores. Serve over ice in a tall glass and decorate with slivers of red cabbage, if liked.

Makes 200 ml (7 fl oz)

Nutritional Values

- Kcals 250
- Vitamin A 49523 iu
- Vitamin C 70 mg
- Potassium 1159 mg
- Selenium 3.79 mcg

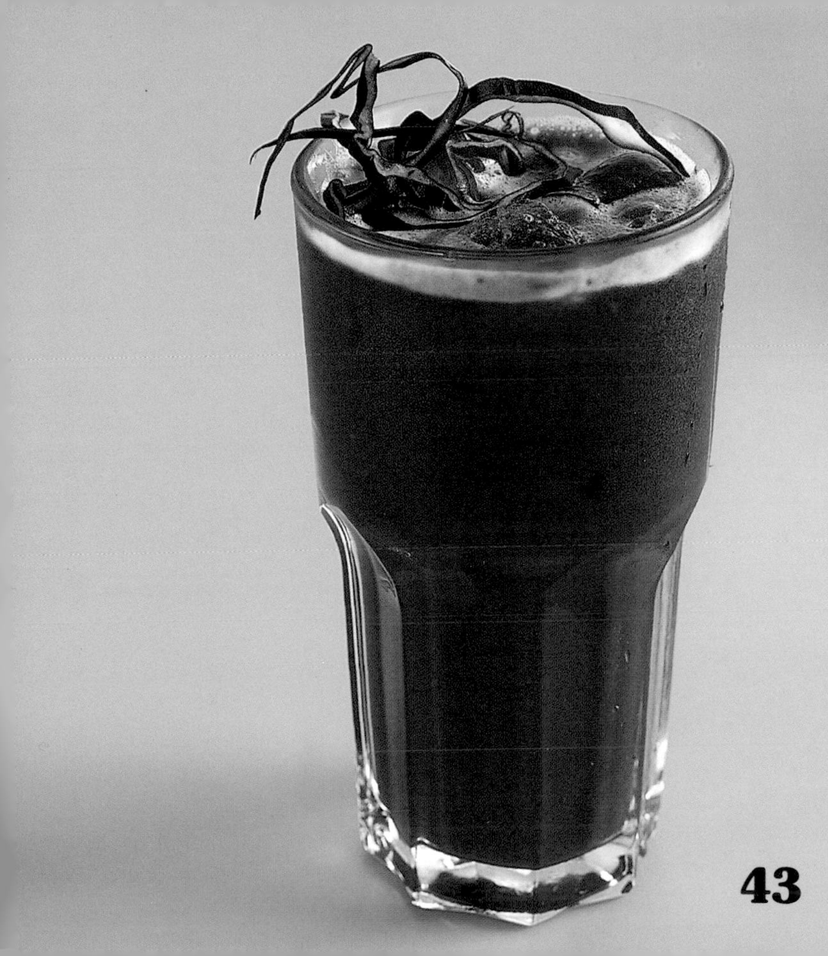

43

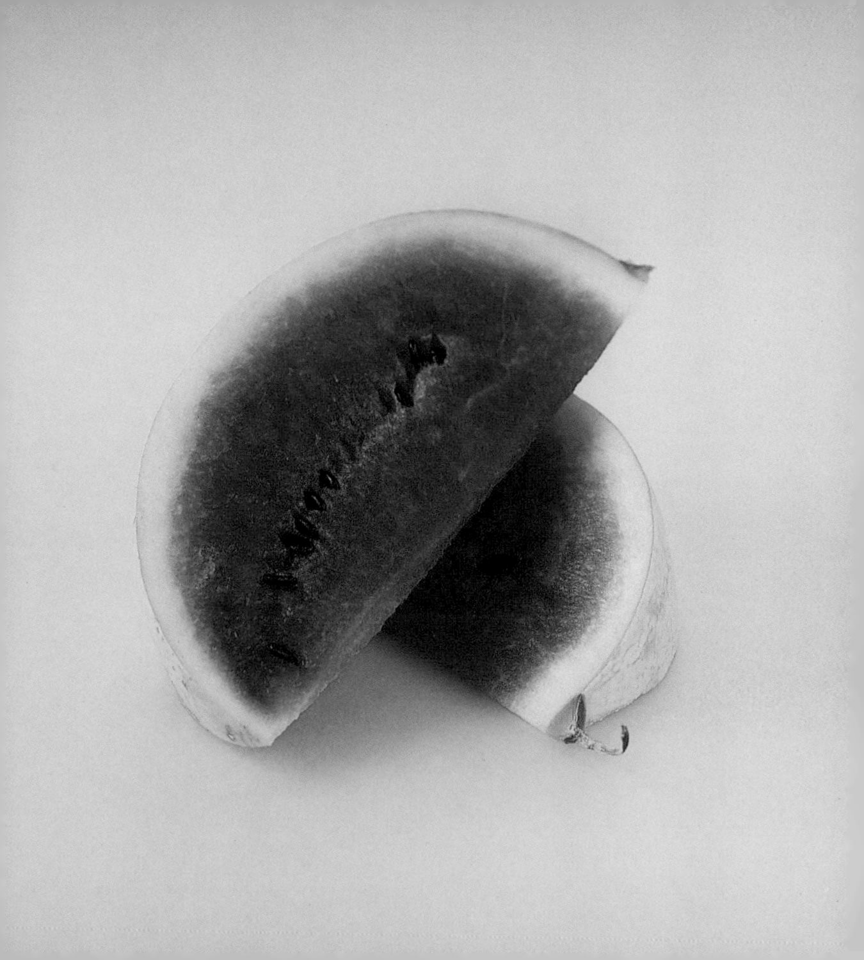

regenerate

Pineapple and grapes are powerful detox fruits and provide a boost of blood sugar, while lettuce and celery both help regenerate the liver and lymph system and aid digestion. All four ingredients can help you sleep.

sleep tight

125 g (4 oz) pineapple
125 g (4 oz) grapes
50 g (2 oz) lettuce
50 g (2 oz) celery

Juice all the ingredients and serve in a tall glass over ice. Decorate with lettuce leaves, if liked.

Makes 200 ml (7 fl oz)

Nutritional Values

- Kcals 167
- Vitamin B6 0.3 mg
- Vitamin C 50 mg
- Magnesium 35.2 mg
- Niacin 1.38 mg
- Tryptophan 4 mg

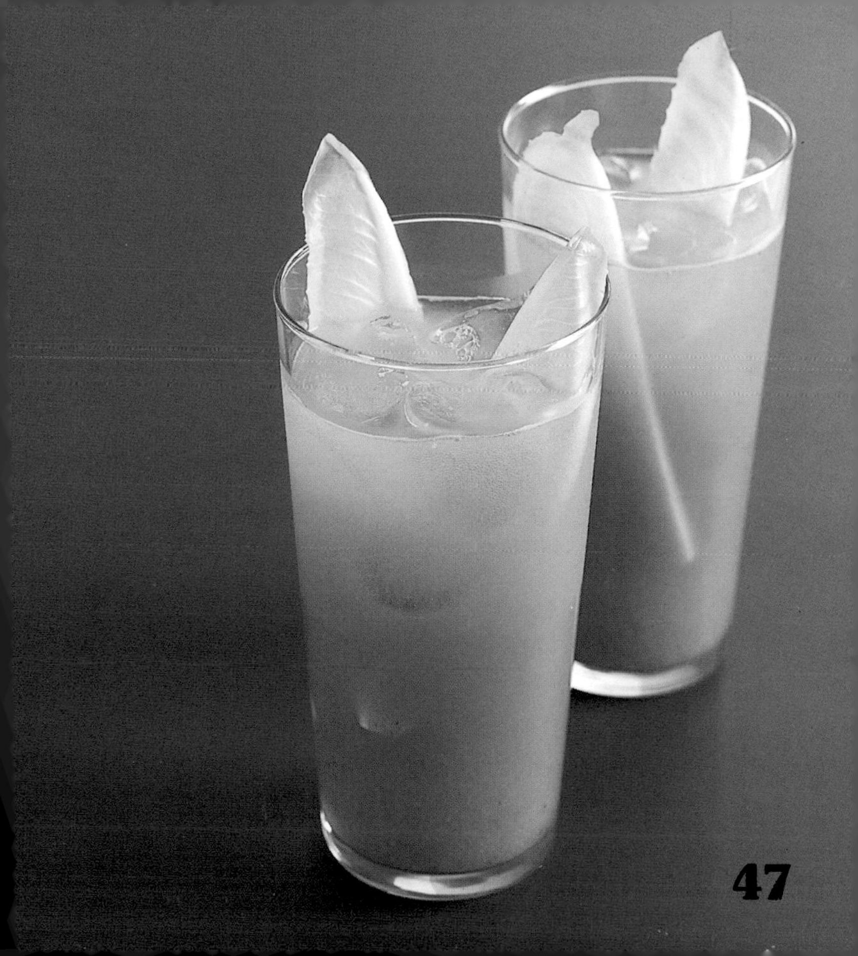

47

This juice cleanses the whole system — blood, kidneys and lymph. All fruits and vegetables with a high water content are useful for helping flush out toxins from the body.

bumpy ride

200 g (7 oz) apple
50 g (2 oz) beetroot
90 g (3 oz) celery

Juice together all the ingredients and serve in a tumbler. Decorate with slices of apple, if liked.
Makes 150 ml (¼ pint)

Nutritional Values

- Kcals 179
- Vitamin A 480 iu
- Vitamin C 23 mg
- Potassium 763 mg
- Magnesium 37 mg

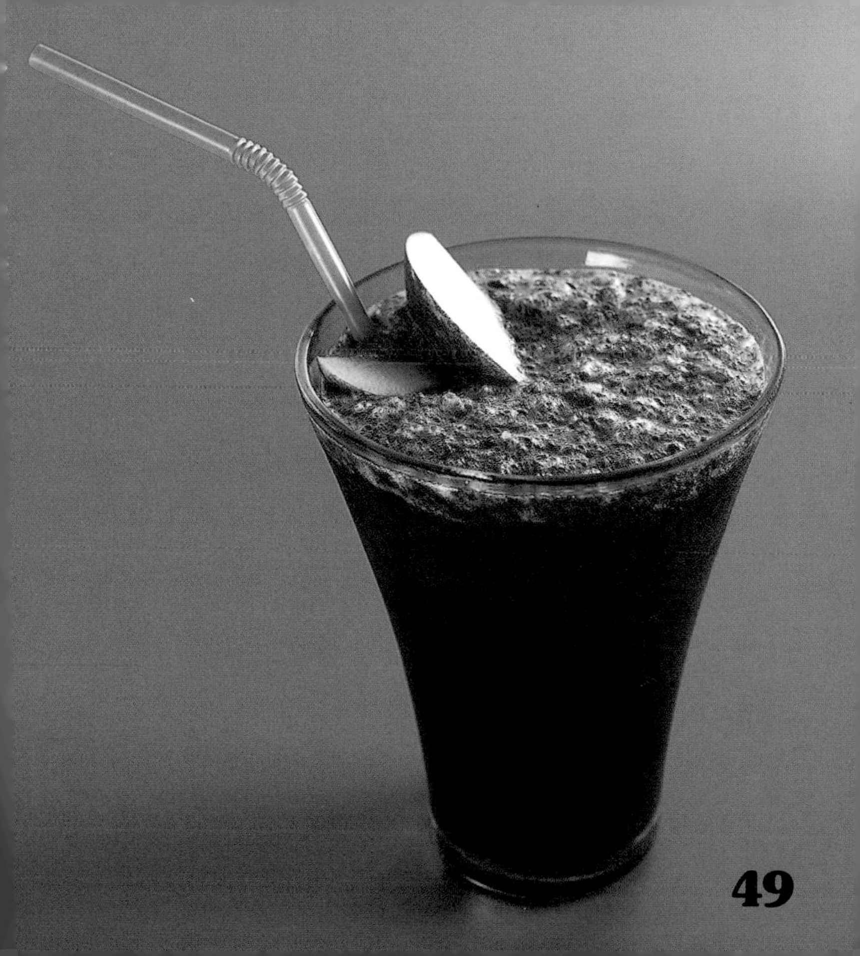

A great detoxing and diuretic fruit, watermelon helps speed up the passage of toxin-carrying fluids through the system.

all systems go

¼ watermelon, about 300 g (10 oz) flesh
2 oranges, peeled

Remove the skin from the watermelon and chop the flesh into even-sized pieces. Juice with the oranges. Pour into a glass and add some ice cubes. Decorate with slices of orange, if liked.

Makes 300 ml (½ pint)

Nutritional Values

- Kcals 200
- Vitamin A 1708 iu
- Vitamin C 170 mg
- Potassium 846 mg
- Iron 1.2 mg
- Calcium 162 mg

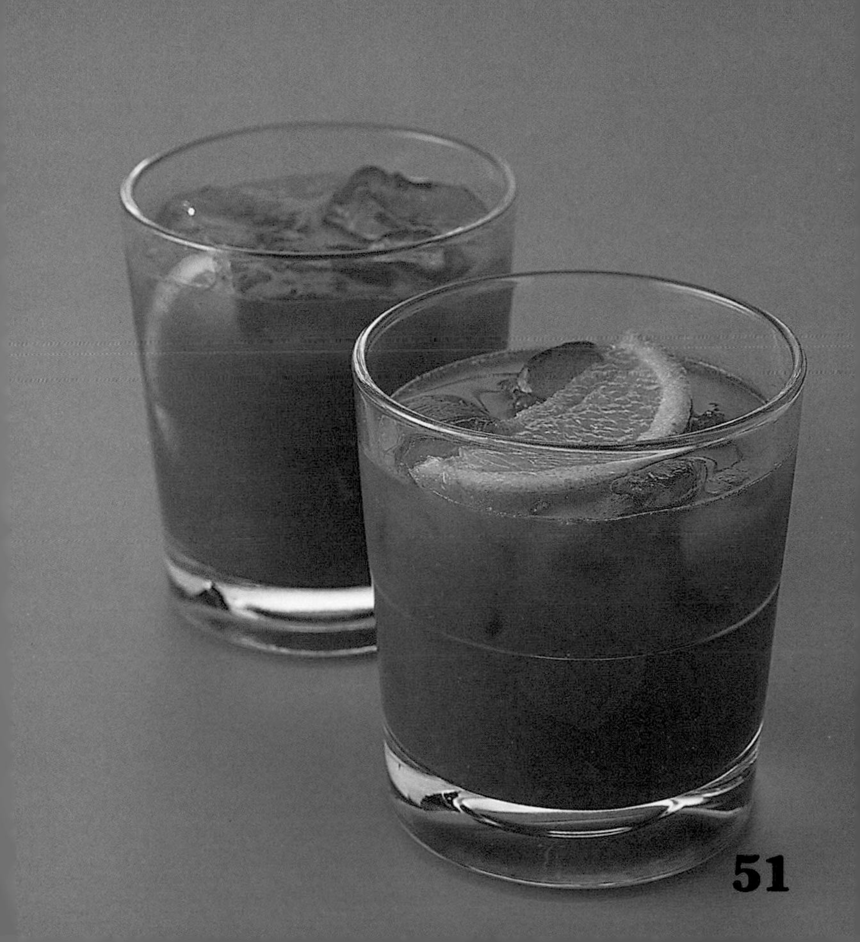

High in fructose, this really flavoursome drink provides instant energy. Pineapple, mango and grapes are fruits with particular detox powers. Both pineapple and mango contain the enzyme bromelin, which helps to produce acids that destroy bad bacteria in the gut, encourage the growth of 'good' bacteria important for digestion, and support tissue repair. Mango also contains the enzyme papain, which helps to break down protein wastes. Grapes help to cleanse the liver and kidneys.

pure cure

100 g (3½ oz) pineapple
100 g (3½ oz) grapes
100 g (3½ oz) orange segments
100 g (3½ oz) apple
100 g (3½ oz) mango flesh
100 g (3½ oz) peeled banana

Juice the pineapple, grapes, orange and apple. Whizz in a blender with the mango, banana and a couple of ice cubes for a super sweet smoothie. Serve decorated with chopped mint and slices of orange, if liked.

Makes 400 ml (14 fl oz)

Nutritional Values

- Kcals 383
- Vitamin A 4631 iu
- Vitamin C 121 mg
- Selenium 3.3 mcg

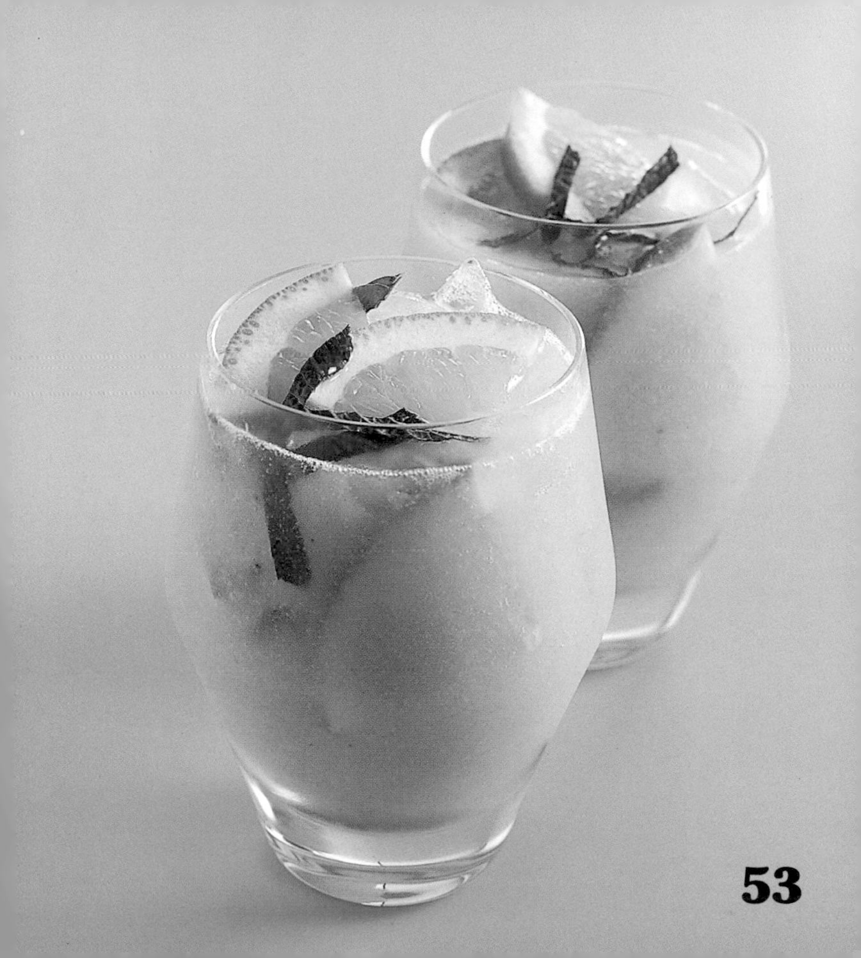

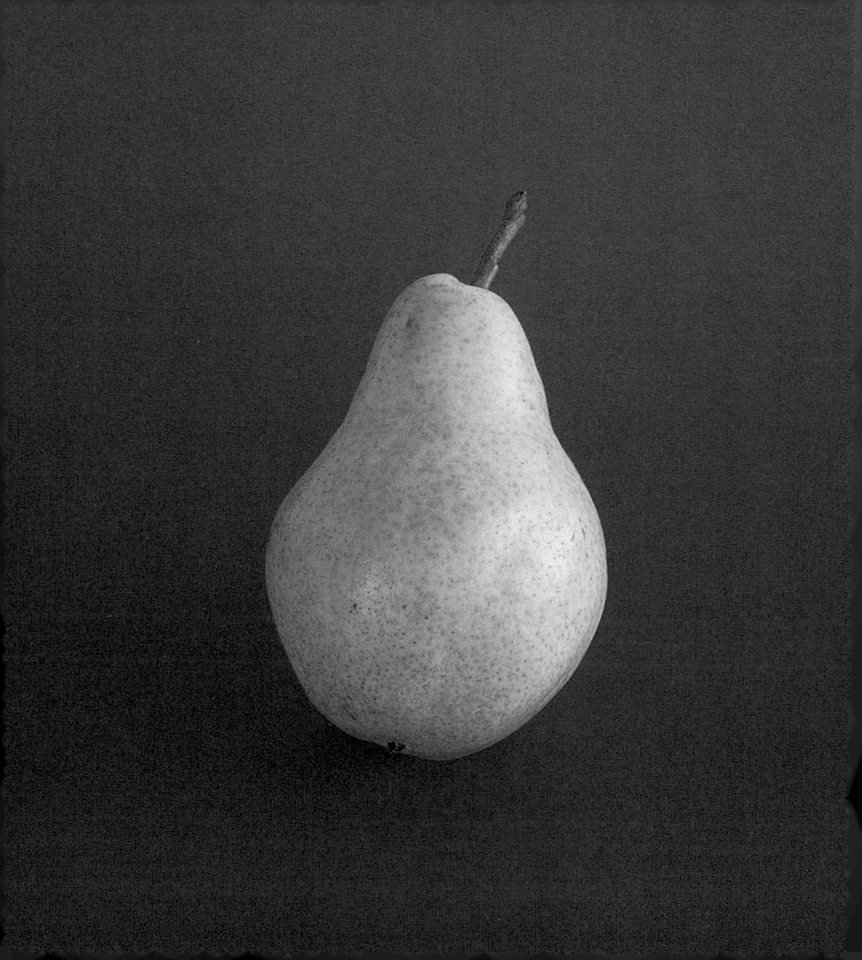

purify

An excellent detoxifier, this juice will prevent the build-up of toxins in your system, which leads to sluggish metabolism, low energy and possibly even serious illnesses. Carrots, lettuce, spinach and celery all work to regenerate the liver and lymph system and aid digestion. Parsley is good for kidney stones, making it the ideal addition to the juice.

squeaky green

175 g (6 oz) carrot
90 g (3 oz) celery
100 g (3½ oz) spinach
100 g (3½ oz) lettuce
25 g (1 oz) parsley

Juice the ingredients and whizz in a blender with a couple of ice cubes. Decorate with sprigs of parsley, if liked.
Makes 200 ml (7 fl oz)

Nutritional Values

- Kcals 137
- Vitamin A 60393 iu
- Vitamin C 120 mg
- Potassium 1855 mg
- Magnesium 138 mg

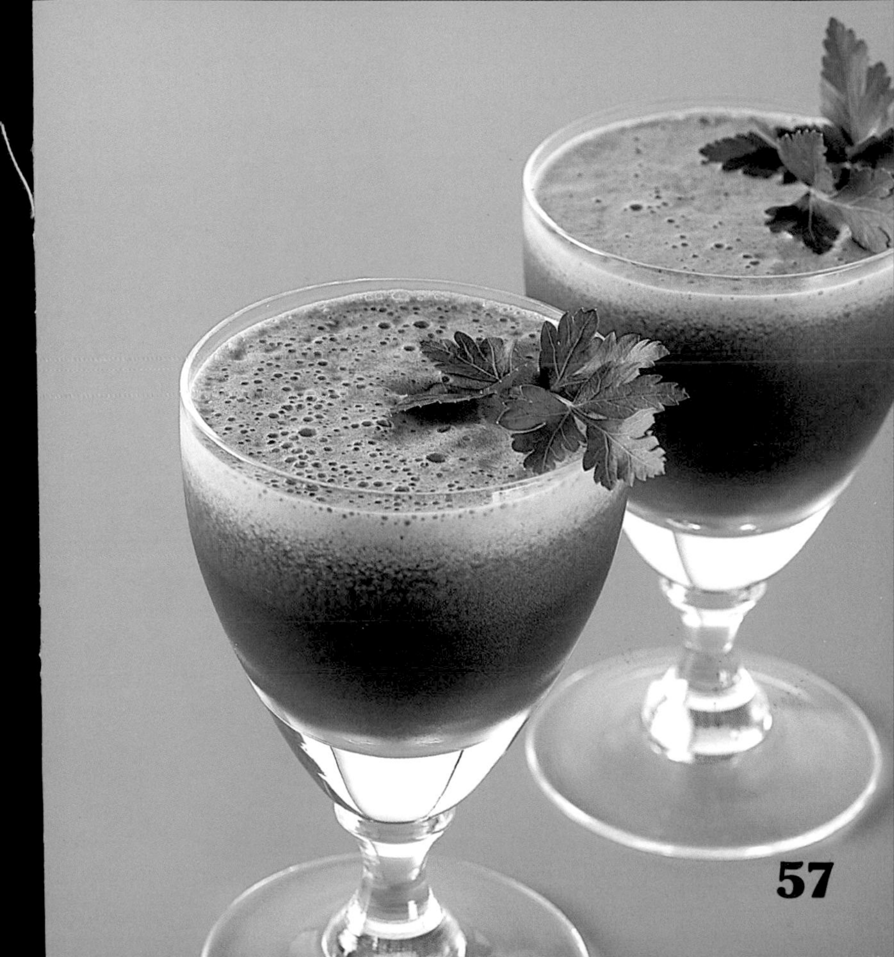
57

Fennel has particularly good detox powers. It also helps to improve digestion and prevent flatulence. Carrots and celery both help the detox process. Available as a powder, spirulina is a form of chlorophyll from the blue-green algae family, which has good energizing properties. In addition, it contains phenylalanine, which suppresses the appetite.

ginger spice

300 g (10 oz) carrot
50 g (2 oz) fennel
75 g (3 oz) celery
2.5 cm (1 inch) cube of fresh root ginger, roughly chopped
1 tablespoon spirulina (optional)

Juice the first four ingredients and serve over ice. Stir in the spirulina, if using. If liked, decorate with strips of fennel and fennel fronds.

Makes 200 ml (7 fl oz)

Nutritional Values

- Kcals 183
- Vitamin A 84600 iu
- Vitamin C 43 mg
- Potassium 1627 mg
- Magnesium 80 mg

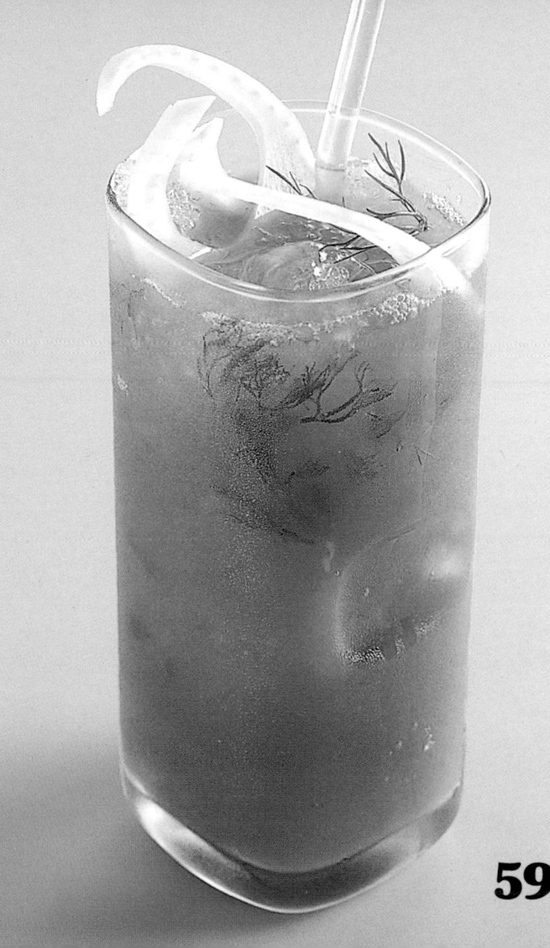

This juice contains potassium, phosphorus and chlorine, all of which are good for skin eruptions. Potato juice is not particularly palatable on its own but is an excellent detoxifier. Radishes are also good for detoxification, while the cucumber flushes out the kidneys.

cucumber cleanser

100 g (3½ oz) potato
100 g (3½ oz) radish
100 g (3½ oz) carrot
100 g (3½ oz) cucumber

Juice the ingredients together and whizz in a blender with a couple of ice cubes. Serve in a tumbler over ice decorated with slices of radish, if liked.
Makes 200 ml (7 fl oz)

Nutritional Values

- Kcals 155
- Vitamin C 56 mg
- Potassium 1242 mg
- Phosphorus 128 mg
- Chlorine 920 mg

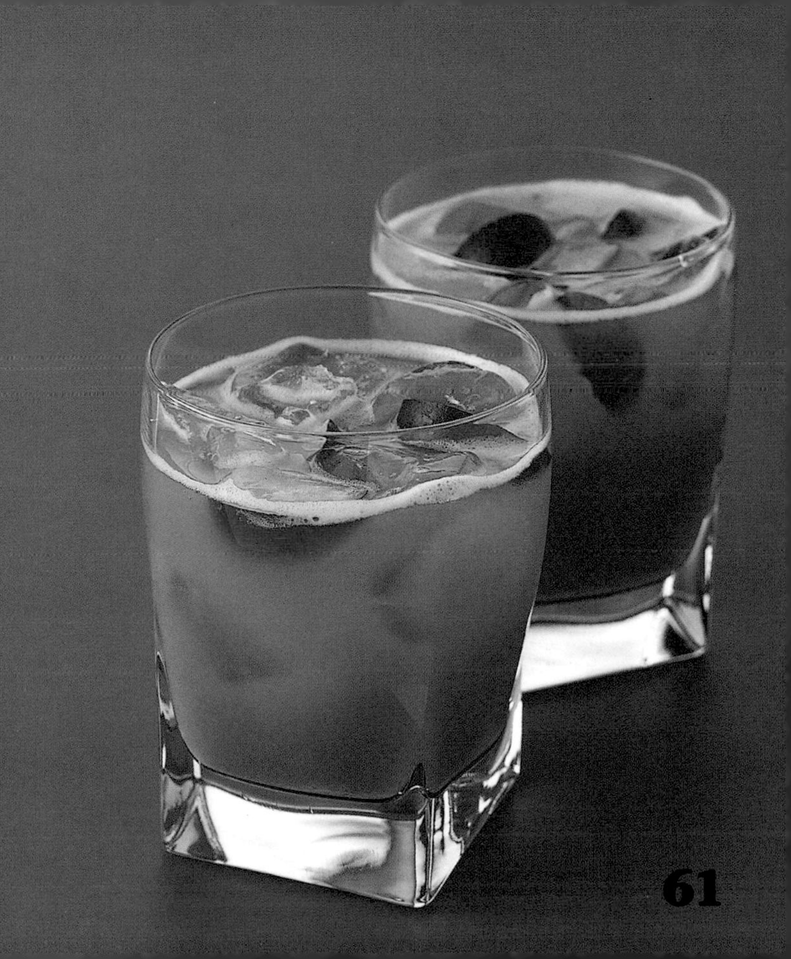
61

Watermelon is the ideal detoxifier, the flesh is packed with beta-carotene and vitamin C. Watermelon juice is so delicious that it's not a chore to drink a glass of this every day. By adding strawberries, you'll be receiving a great boost of vitamin C as well as helping your body fight against bacteria in your system. The juice is also high in zinc and potassium, two great eliminators.

juice boost

200 g (7 oz) watermelon
200 g (7 oz) strawberries

Juice the fruit and whizz in a blender with a couple of ice cubes. Serve decorated with mint sprigs and whole or sliced strawberries, if liked.

Makes 200 ml (7 fl oz)

Nutritional Values

- Kcals 130
- Vitamin A 6562 iu
- Vitamin C 195 mg
- Potassium 950 mg
- Zinc 0.58 mg

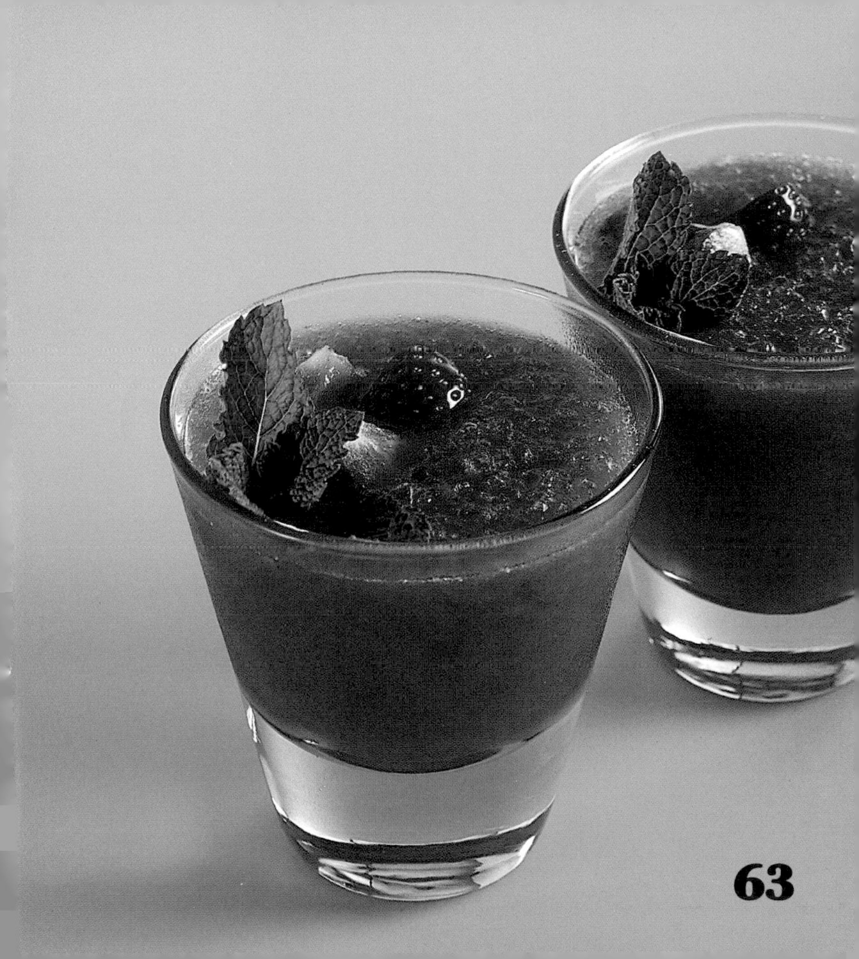
63

index

acknowledgements

The publisher would like to thank The Juicer Company for the loan of The Champion juicer and the Orange X citrus juicer (featured on pages 12 and 13).

The Juicer Company
28 Shambles
York
YO1 7LX
Tel: (01904) 541541
www.thejuicercompany.co.uk

Executive Editor Nicola Hill
Editor Sharon Ashman
Executive Art Editor Geoff Fennell
Designer Sue Michniewicz
Senior Production Controller Jo Sim
Photographer Stephen Conroy
Home Economist David Morgan
Stylist Angela Swaffield